The Golden
Opportunity

How to Prevent Type II Diabetes and It's Life
Threatening Consequences

Rudy Kachmann M.D.

Contents

Preface

ALMOST EVERY MORNING, I HEAD to the Bob Evans restaurant to enjoy an egg white vegetarian omelet with a fruit cup. But it's not every morning that I'm almost brought to tears. Today, I saw a seriously overweight child about 5 years old walk out with his father, who was also clearly overweight. As I sat down, I spied a man in a wheelchair who probably weighed 250 pounds or more, eating a large meal of eggs, sausages, muffins and fried potatoes, along with his wife who was of similar weight and was eating similar foods. After practicing as a physician for more than 44 years in addition to running a wellness show and reading everything on health that I can get my hands on, you can understand why I had tears running down my cheeks. At least 70% of America is in trouble, already suffering from chronic illness or soon to be the victim of a debilitating health condition.

There is great hope, though: All of these people, if properly educated, could prevent, reverse and treat the underlying problems of type 2 diabetes, vascular disease, chronic disease, autoimmune disease, increased chance of cancer and many other illnesses. Unfortunately most people aren't aware of their risk factors or their current health condition.

Hundreds of millions of people have metabolic syndrome, which can lead to type 2 diabetes, vascular disease, hypertension, autoimmune diseases and increased rates of cancer. Many people are completely unaware that this is already occurring. I believe there is a Golden Opportunity here to diagnose, stop and reverse the situation.

In my 44 years of practicing neurosurgery, I found at least one-third of my patients had either pre-diabetes also called diabesity, or type 2 diabetes and many of them had not been properly diagnosed; further, many patients were not aware of the seriousness of their condition.

The main point of this book is to diagnose this large group of patients before their diseases get off the ground.

Generally, patients can be pre-diabetic (diabesity) for 5 to 15 years before their blood sugar ever rises. They may have many other abnormal blood studies as the sugar remained normal. Elevated insulin, which isn't always tested, is the forerunner and marker of pre-diabetes. Elevated insulin inflames 300,000 miles of vascular capillaries, leading to heart attacks, strokes and cancer.

Most people, unfortunately, are not aware that eating the toxic diet of excess fat, salt and sugar inflames their bodies, and is the beginning of many chronic diseases. Their bodies are on fire from food inflammation.

Our genes are not accustomed to this new food that has been introduced in the last 10,000 years, and much more rapidly in the last few decades. Our evolutionary bodies are revolting against this, making us sick.

Our government actually supports this toxic environment through its financial support of corn, wheat, sugar and chemical agriculture, resulting in feedlot animal and fish production. Yes, unfortunately, 90% of the fish we're consuming now comes off the feedlot and not the ocean.

The government is using our tax money and making us sick.

This book is about preventing, reversing and curing these diseases and illnesses, leading to a healthy life and longevity.

Eating all you want of nutrient-dense foods will prevent and reverse horrible conditions such as type 2 diabetes, vascular disease, heart attacks, strokes, hypertension, autoimmune diseases and many types of cancers.

This is not about a diet: It's about eating all you want of healthy, nutrient- dense foods.

This book is about early diagnosis, proper nutrition, a non-diet and proper food selection. And in addition to feeling great, you will also look great!

The Difference between Type 1 and Type 2 Diabetes

TYPE 1 DIABETES IS WHERE you do not make enough insulin to push sugar into the cells for energy. It was considered a juvenile disease, but, it actuality can occur at any age. Some type 2 diabetics can eventually become type 1, and that is the majority of the patients.

type 2 diabetes is due to insulin resistance and the inability of insulin to push sugar into the cell. Ninety percent of diabetics are type 2, and 90% of them may develop type 1 because the pancreas just wears out secreting insulin at a high rate.

Glucose is a sugar and the largest source of energy in the body. Sugar and oxygen chemically react and produce adenosine-triphosphate (ATP) in the mitochondria, or work station, of our body's 70 trillion cells. Without this chemical reaction, we would not be alive. Each of our cells has at least 10,000 mitochondria.

It is very important that we maintain a normal blood sugar. A level too high or too low will have serious consequences. The hormone insulin, glucagon and the liver are all in charge of keeping the blood sugar within reasonable range. When the blood sugar is too low, the liver releases available stored sugar; the liver receives messages from insulin to increase or decrease the amount of sugar; and glucagon is available to stimulate sugar production or breakdown of glucagon, a form of sugar in the muscles and liver. If the system becomes overloaded, the liver will convert glucose or fructose into fat.

Glucagon is the opposite of insulin, and turns on the switch so that fatty acids can be used as an energy source, and it signals the body to increase sugar production.

Type 2 diabetes is preceded by a state of pre-diabetes or diabesity. The whole purpose of this book is to catch those patients at this stage before type 2 diabetes occurs. In pre-diabetes. Insulin levels are elevated for many years, but blood sugars are normal, resulting in great damage to the body. A significant number of patients in the pre-diabetic state develop vascular disease, neuropathy, have heart attacks and strokes, increased rate of cancer, inflammatory disease of the blood vessels and nerves in the body.

10% of type 1 diabetes is usually diagnosed in childhood, but can occur at any age. It is considered an autoimmune disease, where the immune system attacks the pancreas; some cases are thought to be viral in origin.

Patients generally present with weight loss, tremendous thirst and hunger, lack of energy, and episodes of sweating. Blood and urine tests for sugar should be done. Remember, type 2, can lead to type 1 because the pancreas is sick and tired of secreting high amounts of insulin and just plain wears out.

There are other types of diabetes, for example gestational diabetes during pregnancy; a significant number (50%) of these patients go on to have type 2 diabetes in the future. Most of these women are pre-diabetic and the metabolic changes of pregnancy speed things up.

Any pancreatic damage, of course, could cause type 1 diabetes and autoimmune diseases, viral infections, bacterial infections, cancer, and mineral deposits like iron or calcium.

Ninety percent of type 2 diabetics can be prevented, stopped or reversed the majority of the time. Dr. Franklin House from Arizona thinks he can do it in 30 days, some as quickly as a week. Dr. Mark Hyman says it can be done in a week according to a heart study, It's strictly dependent on the type of food you're eating and we'll discuss that in more detail later. Most people have been pre-diabetic for 5 to 15 years before a clear diagnosis is made, which is a very sad situation because the body has already been damaged. This can lead to heart disease and heart attacks, ovarian or uterine cancer, nerve damage or kidney damage. A significant number have impaired vision.

"Early diagnosis" with a two-hour glucose tolerance test is critical; this is essential, otherwise, you can miss the opportunity to avoid the disease altogether. Additional tests of course are important, including the usual fasting blood sugar, HbA 1C, C. reactive protein, homocysteine and lipid profile. The correct diagnosis is critical. Test may need to be repeated for clear diagnosis!

Today I had my hair cut by a young girl at Sweetwater, the great music distribution center where I was trying to arrange a music lesson. Her dad had a stroke at age 50. She's on her way to 180 pounds, with high blood pressure, and she's trying to tell me she's not type 2 diabetic or pre-diabetic. I bet that a provider never checked her insulin level with a two-hour glucose tolerance test. I just know the story too well. I gave her names of books to read as this association can be stopped and possibly reversed. Dr. Dean Ornish proved it in his famous books, as well as Dr. Caldwell Esselstyn.

In summary type 2 diabetes is preceded by a pre-diabetic state where we have a "Golden Opportunity" to stop, prevent and reverse the situation.

Some divide type 2 diabetes into 5 stages:

Stage 1 - insulin resistance (IR) only

Stage 2 - IR, plus hyperinsulinism (HI)

Stage 3 - IR, HI, plus abnormalities in a GTT

Stage 4 - Type 2 diabetes, with high insulin levels

Stage 5 - Type 2 diabetes, with low insulin levels, the end stage

Do you see the problem? If you're diagnosed with stage 5 there are serious consequences.

The disease is prevalent throughout our population and is a great threat to our health and well-being. This is a war worse than anything else attacking our country.

Our evolutionary bodies are not accustomed to what we are eating. We are eating 90% genetically altered, chemically altered, products of fat, salt and sugar and highly processed foods. Our evolutionary history only changes 0.2% every 20,000 years. We greatly changed our food source 10,000 years ago and then through the Industrial Revolution, chemical farming and government support of bad food, all of this is leading to what some people call the United States of Diabesity.

The Awakening

MY DAD HAD A GERMAN deli on 86th Street in Manhattan in the 1940s, '50s and '60s. He worked day and night to provide a good example for this young son; hard work and honesty are the best words to describe my father. We lived within three blocks of the Metropolitan Museum of Art on 81st Street. For the life of me, I still can't understand why I thought that we were poor. I played baseball and tennis in the park almost every day. My mother was a midwife, so me becoming a doctor was a no-brainer. I was told that the day I was born. They handed me a book by a famous German Vietnamese doctor, Dr.Sauerbrook, and that sealed the deal. I remember his picture in a white coat to this day.

The food sold at my dad's deli and most other delis in New York, as well as the gas stations and major food markets today, except for Whole Foods, added a great deal to the obesity problem we have today. They are largely variations of the toxic diet of excess fat, salt and sugar.

It wasn't until the last 20 years or so that I completely realized what was happening with my patients. Medical school then and frankly even today barely teaches proper nutrition to the med students. A medical student told me that she had one hour of study on nutrition and she was a senior.

It is variations of fat, salt and sugar in products that have led to this chronic illness in society. People in general need to have real knowledge about what they're eating. We have 100-150 million people with metabolic syndrome, a syndrome of insulin resistance, hypertension, vascular disease and abnormal fats in their blood. At least 50% of them will develop pre-diabetes and type 2 diabetics. Our food is killing us and we are not aware of it. The government is supplying the bullets. People on food stamps are particularly exposed, look at their obesity rate, close to 90%.

We lead the world in obesity, vascular disease, diabetes, heart attacks and strokes, cancer and autoimmune disease. A third of our teenagers are overweight and guess where that is heading? We even now have obese six-month-old children.

The meat we eat is contaminated with pesticides and herbicides, has been genetically modified, and carries cancer-producing chemicals and growth hormones. This type of farming is destroying our environment with chemicals, pesticides and contaminated water. The government with price supports is making corn, wheat and sugar cheaper to produce. It's a war going on out there, and the enemy is not wearing uniforms that we can easily identify. The government is not supporting the price of vegetables; rather it is supporting the price of animal products that are ruining our health.

Today it's hard to eat a fish from the ocean. Most fish today is farm fed. Read up sometime about CAFOs, concentrated animal feeding organizations. Start off by reading a book called "Slaughterhouse Five" by Kurt Vonnegut, and if you're still eating animal products I would be surprised.

Of course the stressful lives we lead also play a huge part. We're looking for quick fixes to feed the family. We're using food as a tranquilizer. It affects our dopamine and serotonin pathways just like cocaine does. Bad food is as addictive as cocaine or heroin.

In 1961 the Journal of the American Medical Association announced that a vegetarian diet could avoid 97% of coronary artery occlusions. I would say if you ate only 80% that way that would generally work.

Fat, salt and sugar cause insulin resistance, so insulin can't get the sugar into the cell for energy, and the excess insulin is inflaming our whole body, resulting in chronic diseases.

The 40-year-old Framingham heart study in Massachusetts proved that if your triglycerides are less than 150, they give you almost a lifetime guarantee against a heart attack.

Heart attacks, strokes and vascular disease are nutritional diseases for the majority of people. Your family history has little to do with it unless you eat the same diet of fat, salt and sugar. Maybe 10% of people's genes are more threatening than others, but if they eat the right food, that genetic expression generally does not take place.

Dr. Dean Ornish, who has written many famous books, has found that you can even reverse the course of most vascular disease with a truly low-fat diet, largely a plant-based diet. I'm ashamed to say the medical community has largely ignored that information because prevention is not at the top of their list.

The China Study by Dr. Colin Campbell also proves the relationship of heart disease, strokes, diabetes, hypertension, cancer and autoimmune diseases to what you eat. He studied many different villages in China with different eating patterns and found striking results when it comes to food and health.

I recommend books written by Dr. Joel Fuhrman and Dr. Colin Campbell, Dr. Neil Barnard, Dr. McDougall, Dr. Pritikin, Dr. Mark Hyman, Dr. Franklin House, Dr. Richard Johnson, Dr. Dean Ornish, and Dr. Robert Lustig which offer great advice, science and recipes.

A Japanese study found a fourfold increase in breast cancer rates in meat eaters. A cancer specialist recently told me that uterine cancer is 70% related to poor diet. About 30 to 40% of breast cancer is related to obesity. Most women have not been told that, which is shameful. The pink ribbons are not going to solve this problem but proper diet and exercise teaching could help a lot.

Most people think chicken is a health food, however, it's about 30% fat, which carries cholesterol and many chemicals.

Many of our foods are contaminated with viruses, bacteria and chemicals. Most fish served to you comes from a farm pond, a feedlot. They will use leftover products from the slaughter of beef and chicken; you should see the pond they're living in.

According to the Government Accountability Project, many chickens are covered with feces, bile and spoiled food. Many chickens, turkeys and ducks have no bone structure because they grew up in little cages where they couldn't spread their wings. Organic means they open the front door and the back door and never let them out.

Next time you go to a restaurant, ask the waiter whether their fish came from a pond, a feedlot or from the ocean. You might be surprised at the answer. Farm-fed fish is filled with (Arachidonic acid) AA that can cause inflammation.

At my country club the other day, none of the fish on the menu came from the ocean. Interestingly, about 30% of fish has been found to be mis-labeled.

What about Omega 3 fatty acids, the good fat we need and want because it is anti-inflammatory and healing? Good sources include soy products, flaxseeds, olive oil, walnut oils and vegetables. Fish is not the only source; it can also be contaminated with viruses, lead and mercury.

Take a close look at yourself and your family. Many of my patients over the past four-and-half decades have been completely unaware of what's going on in their bodies. Most Americans at age 60 have at least one chronic disease, which could likely be avoided with greater knowledge about food, exercise, stress reduction and spirituality.

Metabolic Syndrome

METABOLIC SYNDROME IS ALSO CALLED insulin resistance syndrome" or Syndrome X. To make a diagnosis, you need to consider a number of risk factors.

In 2005, the American Heart Association and the National Heart, Lung and Blood Institute published the following risk profile for metabolic syndrome:
- Is your HDL number below 40 for men or below 50 for women?
- Are your triglycerides over 150?
- Is your waist size 35 inches or above for women, or 40 inches or above for men?
- Are you a pre-diabetic or diabetic, with fasting glucose 100 or greater?
- Is your blood pressure consistently 130/85 or greater?

Metabolic syndrome is a combination of multiple cardiac risk factors believed to be a product of insulin resistance. Our cells, protected by receptors, control which nutrients are allowed in. If these receptors on the cells are made sticky, then the insulin cannot transport the sugar into the cell and that is what we called insulin resistance.

Unfortunately, these receptors can become resistant to insulin's action, probably as a result of weight gain and physical inactivity. This scenario, if repeated over time, is thought to trigger a series of metabolic maladies culminating in metabolic syndrome. The condition directly damages the coronary arteries, causing the build-up of plaque and promoting blood clots.

Metabolic syndrome affects more than 75 million Americans. It was originally described by Dr. Gerald M. Raven at Stanford University and he called it Syndrome X. Insulin resistance is at the crossroads of this X with obesity, hypertension, abnormal blood fats and high triglycerides being the four legs.

Frankly, you can generally look at a person and guess whether they have metabolic syndrome by their body size. Actually, about 20% of people with metabolic syndrome or syndrome X are of normal weight but their blood factors are abnormal. So it is important to get your lipid profile, CRP, and other indicators of inflammation. Many providers use only two or three of these indicators to make a diagnosis. This improves the chances of reversing the condition.

Insulin resistance is the key to the diagnosis. Insulin is one of the body's most powerful hormones, a class of chemicals that cause enormous physiological changes. It can cause inflammation of the joints that lead to arthritis and also can cause sodium retention in our body, resulting in hypertension, and type 2 diabetes, Ca, dementia, etc.

Many people walking around with metabolic syndrome have been totally undiagnosed. This is extremely serious because with proper treatment, they could prevent the development of serious chronic diseases and avoid a lot of suffering, medical costs and possibly disability and death. Many go blind, need to have transplants and even have extremities amputated. There is a much higher rate of dementia and Alzheimer's disease also among these patients.

It is my opinion and the opinion of many others that the most accurate test to determine insulin resistance is the two-hour glucose tolerance test. But it is critical to test blood sugar as well as the serum insulin. Stage one is insulin resistance. Also, I suggest the HbA 1C but it may be normal because the blood sugar was not elevated. It is critical to know your insulin level, which many times is forgotten and not commonly ordered.

The shape of the body can also give you clues as to insulin resistance in metabolic syndrome. Apple shape is more threatening than pear-shaped, since this type of person generally has more fat inside the liver, pancreas or intestines. Subcutaneous fat is not as threatening, as seen in a pear-shaped individual.

A person under a lot of stress would tend to have a big belly because of steroids, specifically cortisol, which like to deposit fat there; that also is a sign of insulin resistance and pre-diabetes or diabetes.

Very low-density cholesterol (VLDLDL) is the most dangerous of the fats because it can inflame your arteries and damage the endothelium, resulting in invasion of the endothelium by fat deposits.

Insulin also turns on the sympathetic nervous system, your stress response system, resulting in elevation of the blood pressure, your general stress reaction and also increased sugar and fat metabolism.

In 1997 the federal government recommended that all people should be checked for diabetes by age 45. It's my opinion that a lot of these diabetic patients are being missed because they don't get the proper tests.

A national survey revealed in 1998 that the baby boomers are being diagnosed with pre-diabetes at age 37. In 1998 the CDC recommended that every adult be checked for diabetes by age 25. I say let's try age 15 or less because of the great number of obese teenagers.

The earlier we make a diagnosis, the sooner we can begin to avoid a lot of chronic disease; we could turn this into the healthiest nation in the world and improve our ranking of 37 according to the World Health Organization at this time.

Pre-diabetes

THERE ARE ABOUT 75-125 MILLION pre-diabetics in this country, and a significant number are children. Vascular disease starts at age 2 as proven by autopsies on children. These patients are painting their 300,000 miles of capillaries with inflammation and cholesterol deposits which can lead to blindness, amputations, renal transplants, heart attacks and strokes. This population also has a much higher rate of cancer: 75% of uterine cancers are based on obesity, 30 to 40% of breast cancers are related to obesity.

Right now these pre-diabetics are looking pretty good, some are even of normal weight, some are slightly overweight and a significant number may be clearly obese.

An unannounced heart attack is not uncommon; this is usually the event that enters the person into the primary healthcare system and the diagnosis of diabetes.

10% of patients will have a family history of heart attack, stroke, hypertension and diabetes at a young age, but it is much more likely what you're eating and not your family history that determine your future.

The other day I was working out at Planet Fitness. A young man was standing at the desk and mentioned that his dad had by-pass surgery yesterday. I asked him if he ever had his blood work checked, since his father had his problem for a few years now; he said no -- a major mistake. In spite of his low body mass index, we don't know the biometrics of his body, which can be a real problem. I wrote out the necessary tests he should get fairly soon. For all we know he has very abnormal blood studies. His dad's problem didn't start yesterday, it started decades ago.

Prevention is the key.

What are signs of pre-diabetes?
- Hypertension
- Family history
- Weight gain-obesity (especially waist circumference)
- Lack of energy
- Numbness in the arms or legs
- Memory loss
- Apple shape or pot belly
- Visual problems
- Skin rashes
- Abnormal lipids
- Elevated CRP
- Abnormal 2-hour glucose tolerance test
- Elevated insulin level

I think people should be screened for pre-diabetes at a very young age if we're going to catch them all. The CDC recommends 25 years of age but I'm recommending 10-15 years of age if we're going to have some impact on the serious health problems in this nation.

Routine blood work should include, lipid profile and CRP, (C-reactive protein), homocysteine level, serum fibrinogen level, HbA 1C, fasting blood sugar and a 2 hour glucose tolerance test and with a fasting 2 hour serum insulin. The serum insulin is critical to this test, and that's what many people miss.

Hemoglobin is a protein found in the red blood cells that attaches itself to oxygen and sugar, and when you run the tests, you get a good look at the blood sugar but not the serum insulin. The serum insulin will rise before the elevation of the blood sugar, by many years and that is the 'Golden Opportunity" for corrective action. If you are pre-diabetic, you need to take action quickly because of the potential complications. They also need to know your lipid profile, types of fat you have, low-density, high density and whether you have a small or large fat particles which makes a difference in the rate of vascular disease.

I suggest:
- Triglycerides less than 150
- LDL less than 70
- HDL greater than 60 for females
- HDL greater than 50 for males
- BS<100
- CRP<1
- VLDLDL< 500 particles
- Triglyceride ratio / HDL<2

Other risk factors include family history, blood pressure and especially activity level. Couch potatoes are more likely to have insulin resistance. An apple shape can almost guarantee it.

The American College of Endocrine Task Force on Prevention of Diabetes recommends a blood pressure of about 130/80. Your health risk assessment and your biometrics tell the story very well. Remember even normal weight people can have pre-diabetes and need their blood work checked. If you're over 60, the most recent B.P. recommendation is 150/90.

Pre-Diabetes and Overweight Kids

THIRTY TO 40 YEARS AGO pre-diabetes in a child was rare.

Now we see even type 2 diabetics as teenagers. Some children are obese at just six months. The mother's nutrition during pregnancy is critical. The mother's diet will determine the metabolism of her child through epi-genetics. Now we're seeing type 2 diabetics as teenagers and adults in there 20s and 30s and up; the earlier the pre-diabetic is diagnosed and treatment occurs, the easier it is to reverse. Many of our children are couch potatoes today: texting, using the Internet, watching TV while eating empty calories, which affects their dopamine circuitry.

Measure your waist and hips, because BMI is important to pre-diabetes but it is not the last word. The fat in your organs tell the real story and this may not be easy to diagnose. Your family doctor or pediatrician needs to be a wellness doctor.

Your weight is the main factor you have in controlling pre-diabetes. Remember some people have pre-diabetes with a normal weight, so you need to know your lipid profile; CRP is critical at any age, it indicates inflammation in your body.

BMI is different for different ethnic and racial groups. A BMI of 18.5-24.9 is considered healthy for the white population. Generally, with the black population, you can add five points and a normal BMI for them may be 35. The Asian population's BMI is five points below 25. A BMI over 40 is considered morbidly obese. What is interesting is that a 5 to 10% weight loss many times can reverse pre-diabetes or diabetes type 2. The best advice is to get a normal BMI as quickly as you can.

Besides, an overall reduction in weight makes you look good and feel better; you will get sick less often and avoid major diseases.

Remember 90% of the time type 2 diabetes leads to type 1. Then you'll need shots and begin heading towards end-stage kidney disease with its usual complications.

Prevention and cure of pre-diabetes is the answer. Many people are pre-diabetic 10 to 15 years before a proper diagnosis is made. Millions of people are literally walking time bombs. Our bodies and organs are being invaded by fat, salt and sugar from fast food restaurants; government support of foods is killing us; stress is the most common cause of our overeating and we crave the feel-good hormones of dopamine and serotonin supplied by fat, salt and sugar.

Fiber: Your friend

FAST FOOD RESTAURANTS SELL FOOD without fiber. They want quick results. They want you to feel the serotonin and dopamine of sugar and fat products within seconds. Fiber delays digestion and that is not what they are interested in.

If you're having a weight problem and especially trying to get over some chronic disease like vascular disease, type 2 diabetes, arthritis, heart issues, sleep apnea, autoimmune disease or cancer, pay attention to the amount of fiber you eat every day.

What is fiber? Fiber is what makes your food more difficult to chew. Animal meat does not have fiber. Plants have fiber. Fiber comes as soluble or non-soluble. The non-soluble is made from polysaccharides, not sugar; soluble fiber is made from complex sugar chains. Fiber is also known as roughage or bulk and it's a secret weapon in our nutrition story. Many people are not aware or informed about it. Dr. Robert Lustig in his famous book "Fat Chance" considers fiber "half the antidote" for weight loss.

Fiber blocks the absorption of a lot of bad fats, simple sugars, processed foods and more. About 30% of the high fiber foods we eat will pass in the stool undigested. We could lose about 30% of all of our ingested calories passively in the feces and as a result lose weight and improve our metabolism.

Because we eat a lot of low-fiber food and animal products, many people in our society don't get enough fiber in their diet.

Dietitians recommend 14 grams of fiber per 1,000 calories with a total of about 25 grams daily.

Soluble fiber is found in fruits and vegetables. Non-soluble fiber is found in stems of plants. The soluble fiber slows digestion, and is fermented by bacteria into gases. Insoluble fiber is made from polysaccharides, such as cellulose, the stringy stuff in celery.

Soluble fiber absorbs water, and good examples are oatmeal, lentils, apples, oranges, pears, oat bran, strawberries, flaxseeds, beans, dried peas, blueberries, cucumbers and carrots. Insoluble fiber does not absorb water and examples are whole wheat, whole grains, wheat bran, corn, brain, seeds, nuts, barley, couscous, brown rice, zucchini, celery, broccoli, cabbage, onions, tomatoes, celery, cucumbers, green beans, dark leafy vegetables, fruit and root vegetable skins.

Metabolically, the two together are unbeatable. The insoluble fiber forms a latticework for the soluble fiber to sit on, while the soluble fiber bridges the gaps in the latticework to maintain its integrity. Inhibiting the rate of flux from the intestines into the bloodstream is a good thing. It gives the liver a chance to fully metabolize what's going on, so there's no overflow. Besides, it keeps a lot of the bad food out. Unfortunately, the majority of foods we are consuming today lack fiber of any sort. Fast food restaurants specialize in that. Refined grains are stripped of both the bran, the outside covering and the germ, the process of milling. This gives a finer texture and extends shelf life while taking out various micronutrients, vitamins and minerals, and phytochemicals. Refined rice is higher on the glycemic index than brown rice.

The USDA doesn't consider fiber an essential nutrient, so it is ignored, a major mistake leading to our obesity crisis. Thousands of years ago, we ate a very high fiber diet and we were a lot healthier.

Last night I was having dinner at an outdoor restaurant on a beautiful fall Indiana evening.

My appetizer was made from celery sticks, pepper sticks, and asparagus, cucumber and broccoli. I then dipped it in hummus, full of fiber and protein. A perfect appetizer because it was delicious, full of vitamins, minerals, phytochemicals and fiber. The increased fiber satisfied my gut and prevented me from eating any extra calories.

When you eat food with significant fiber, you automatically increase your vitamins, minerals and phytochemicals in a mosaic of great nutrition. Your metabolism will improve quickly and speed up. Your type 2 diabetes will disappear pretty quickly. Dr. Franklin House in "The 30 Day Miracle" claims he can get rid of your type 2 diabetes 90% of time in about 30 days and I believe him. Other good books to read would be by Dr. Caldwell Esselstyn, Dr. Dean Ornish, Dr. Joel Fuhrman, Dr. Neal Barnard and Dr. Mike McDougall. Incidentally, my book "The Secret of the Non-diet and Reversing type 2 Diabetes" is a summary of the information I've learned from these books, other books and many medical papers as well as 44 years of seeing patients.

Fiber is a true friend.

Increasing your fiber by eating beans, vegetables and many other plant foods will greatly improve your health.

High Fructose Corn Syrup (HFCS)

THE "BLISS POINT" FOR PLAIN old sugar as you might suspect has been found by the food manufacturers: It's 26% for adults, and 36% for children. In other words, as adults, if 26% of our food is sugar and it would still be palatable. Sales were becoming stagnant so the industry needed something sweeter and especially cheaper.

In 1970 the Japanese invented high fructose corn syrup (HFCS). It is now made from government-supported corn; the sugar from corn syrup is modified with an enzyme and that makes it a lot sweeter and cheaper. Unfortunately, it's metabolized differently, and was placed in soft drinks and a lot of other foods. Some restrictions have been made in certain states to restrict the sale because of health hazards. Then again, it is not that different from regular sucrose, which is 50% of glucose and 50% sucrose. Certainly, Dr. Robert Lustig, a pediatric endocrinologist, thinks so and put that on his "YouTube DVD" and his great book called "Fat Chance." He hit the nail on the head as to the cause of our obesity epidemic.

It is my opinion, well supported in the literature and my books plus 44 years of experience, that sugar is a toxin that makes us sick and fructose is the "Evil Twin". Remember sucrose and table sugar is 50% glucose and 50% fructose.

Sugar is both a carbohydrate and a fat and I will prove it to you.

Sugar is bar none the most successful food additive.

Now, because of fructose corn syrup, which is so much cheaper, sugar in some form is found in 80% of our 60,000 food products.

Sugar is made from 50% glucose and 50% fructose. It's fructose that makes it sweet, that is the molecule we want. It's fructose that causes metabolic syndrome and accompanying diseases. The changes occur in the liver because that is where fructose is metabolized.

After digestion, the sugar molecule splits into sucrose and fructose. Fructose goes straight to the liver and is rapidly converted to fat and not used for energy. Of the 50% of the sucrose that is sugar, only 25% goes to the liver versus 80% of the fructose which heads straight for the liver and is converted to low density LDL, the nasty stuff that causes vascular disease. Glucose can replace your glycogen stores, your sugar stores that are used widely for exercise and daily activity.

Americans consume 150 pounds of sugar yearly, 6.5 ounces a day. Our consumption has doubled in 30 years. The CDC estimates that Americans consume one can of sweetened drink daily, 5% consume four drinks a day. World consumption has doubled in 50 years.

The American Heart Association recommends only 200 calories from sugar per day and that is being exceeded all over the world.

The fructose corn syrup consumption rate has gone down a bit because of education and the change of some laws in cities like New York. Mayor Michael Bloomberg has done his best but he didn't get everything done that he wanted to do in that direction. Except from fruit because of its fiber, fructose is toxic and is killing a lot of us. Incidentally, the fructose in fruit is metabolically no different!

Orange juice is worse than fructose corn syrup: In just one eight-ounce glass, there is nearly two grams of fructose. The same thing goes with soda.

All sweets have fructose, including white sugar, beans, table sugar, honey, brown sugar, etc.

Sugar stimulates our serotonin and dopamine circuitry and makes us feel good quickly. A significant number of us, including newborns, are addicted to sugar. The bigger you are, the more likely that has occurred; you may not even be aware of it. Sugary drinks account for 50% of the obesity in the United States and the world over. Diet drinks aren't much better because they have a sweet taste that encourages people to eat more sugary foods and the obesity epidemic continues.

Certainly, if you're an athlete in the middle of a major event and drinking sugary drinks, you would probably get away with it because you are using them up as energy very quickly, but the rest of us watching the race will gain weight quickly although fructose is not metabolized quickly.

When the fructose is metabolized in the liver and causes insulin resistance, it does not turn off our appetite or signal the brain that we have enough energy and so it leads to weight gain. That is because of leptin and insulin resistance.

Our bodies have not adjusted to the sugary glut and we gain weight instead and develop insulin resistance, type 2 diabetes and many other chronic illnesses.

As already mentioned, sugar is added to about 80% of our 60,000 foods and we don't even notice it, so reading labels becomes important. The government supports the price of sugar, which is making us sick; it supports the price of corn, the source of fructose corn syrup; your own government has declared war on you. The lobbyists for these food companies pass out a lot of money to the politicians whose main concern appears to be to be reelected and your health is irrelevant. They can show us the food plate all they want, but actions speak louder than words. We lead the world in vascular disease, diabetes, cancer and autoimmune disease. Remember the critical worlds: Sugar is 50% fructose, it's a carbohydrate and a fat and that's what's killing us. Read your labels, talk to the waiter, always ask where the food came from. You need to be an informed consumer or you'll surely get sick.

Protein
(of Prime Importance)

IF YOU UNDERSTAND THE PHYSIOLOGY of protein, then proper food selection is easy. Knowing the difference between plant and animal protein is life saving and will help you avoid a lot of the illnesses, cause you to look and feel good, and probably live to be 100.

Protein consists of 20 amino acids and is made from the minerals nitrogen and carbon. Eight of the amino acids are essential; in other words you have to eat them and they cannot be made by the body. Protein is found in your bones, skin, hormones, cartilage, teeth, nails, hair and muscles.

In 1988 the Academy of Nutrition and Dietetics said plant protein could meet the nutritional requirements of all adults and children when eating a variety of foods. Plants provide all the necessary amino acids.

This certainly was a very important statement and contradicts a lot of false information out there. A lot of people think you need to eat animal protein to get all the necessary protein for growth and that is just plain wrong.

Nitrogen, the principal chemical of protein, was discovered in 1839. It was the most sacred of nutrients at that time. Most people thought only animal meats had protein.

In 1960, the UN declared an international protein deficiency epidemic. In 1970 they admitted they had been wrong. As a result there has been great confusion over the following:

- What are the best sources of protein?
- How much protein should we consume?
- Is plant protein as good as animal protein?
- Is it necessary to combine certain foods to get all the protein we need?
- Is it necessary to take certain protein supplements?
- Where do vegetarians get their protein?
- Do vegetarian children grow properly?

It didn't help that in 1970 Dr. Lappe published a book called "A Diet for Our Planet" that claimed that only animal protein supplied the amino acids we need. A decade later she published another book stating she had been wrong.

In the 1900s, many wealthy people ate a high animal protein diet; the poor ate more of a plant diet. The rich became sick and the poor were healthier, contrary to what we are seeing today. In 1900 Dr. Max Rubles stated we needed only 50 grams of protein daily. Frankly, this is a pretty accurate figure. His student Dr. Atwater recommended 125 grams, but it was too much and found to be hard on the liver and kidneys that had to metabolize and then excrete it. The medical talk in the 1960s and '70s was about the protein gap.

Dr. Colin Campbell from Cornell University along with a Chinese epidemiologist and a British statistician studied the diet of the Chinese in many different cities. He correlated what people ate and what illnesses and diseases they developed and then published a very famous book called "The China study."

The people that were eating largely a plant-based diet were very healthy and did not develop a lot of the Western diseases. The people who ate processed food and a lot of animal products are the ones who develop diabetes, heart disease, strokes increased cancer rates, etc. He found a clear relationship between high-protein meat diets and the diseases of hypertension, heart disease, vascular disease, heart attacks, cancer, autoimmune disease, etc.

What is animal meat composed of? Saturated fat, cancer-causing blood products, insulin growth factor, cholesterol, etc. Plant protein is not accompanied by any of these chemicals. There's no cholesterol in plants.

Remember, even meat with all visible fat removed is still 30 to 40% fat.

Plants have all the essential amino acids without the fat, no cholesterol, and offer 14 vitamins, 25 minerals, and 25,000 phytochemicals. It is the interaction of these vitamins, minerals and phytochemicals that leads to good health.

Besides if you follow what goes on in "CAFOs" or concentrated animal feeding organizations, you will think twice about eating animal products. If you were to read "The Omnivores Dilemma" or "The Mad Cowboy," they will open your eyes.

A lot of the diet books recommend too many animal products as far as I'm concerned.

What are your protein needs?
- Males - .8-1 g/kilo
- Females - .5-1 g/kilo
- May be higher depending on amount of and type of exercise, 1 to 2 g per kilo
- Average 50 to 60 g daily

Some of these high-protein diets recommend up to 300 grams of protein daily and that can be toxic to your liver and kidneys.

Protein is broken down in the liver; two-thirds of it actually is recycled and you only have to replace one-third of it daily.

Dr. Rip Esselstyn, a fireman who wrote a great book on beef and protein and plant diets, became a successful triathlete. Whole Foods has a great CEO, John Mackey, and the majority of food in those stores is labeled with the nutrient density scores of Dr. Joel Fuhrman. Dr. Mackey also published a famous book called "Conscious Capitalism." You can see he has health-focused customers in his mind besides trying to make a profit. I take my hat off to him. I don't think that the majority of our huge food marketing companies, our government that supports the price of fat, salt and sugar, or our Cattlemen's Association are wearing the same hat.

Who's the biggest and fastest? The plant eaters or the meat eaters? Actually, it's not even a contest. Recently I met a plant-eating gorilla and took a picture with him in the San Diego Zoo. Next time you're there be sure to say hello to my new friend David the silverback gorilla, plant-eating animals live longer too!

Some people claim that we were mainly animal eaters in earlier times. I think they're completely wrong. We have over 20 feet of intestinal bowel, which is seen in plant eaters, while meat eaters have four feet of bowel like the lion. Our genes only change .0045% every 20,000 years. So what do you think? It's quite clear we were mainly plant eaters hundreds of thousands of years ago.

Protein supplementation should only be considered for the most advanced of weightlifters.

Wild game is only 10 to 20% fat. Farm raised animals fed with feed corn are full of inflammatory fats and should be avoided.

The book called "The Paleo Diet" has a great list of low-fat animal meat with fat and protein content. So if you're going to eat some animal meat, which even Dr. Joel Fuhrman would agree with, no more than two times per week or so, choose a high-protein, low-fat version:

- Skinless turkey breast: 94% protein, 5% fat
- Boiled shrimp: 90% protein, 10% fat
- Red snapper: 87% protein, 13% fat.
- Alaskan King crab legs: 85% protein, 15% fat.
- Hot dogs: 14% protein, 83% fat

Are you getting the idea? Most of us would like to eat some meat protein and to have a nice list of high-protein, low-fat foods in mind is a great thing.

Dr. Franklin House wrote a book called the "The 30 Day Miracle" which points out that adults don't need a lot of protein. He points out that a baby doubles its weight in 120 days and certainly mother's milk protein is essential. A rat eats a lot of protein and doubles its weight in 4.5 days. We don't need all that. The meat we are eating is full of pesticides, herbicides, cancer growth factors, angiogenesis factors and it's killing us.

Dr. House states that a plant diet will decrease your triglycerides 100 points in six weeks. He has been running the Lifestyle Institute in Arizona and California for 30 years and I tend to believe him. Before taking medication, you might try the plant diet for two or three months. Dr. House says no long-term study proves that low carbohydrate diets work.

Soy products are high-protein and quite healthy, including tofu and seitan, if not genetically modified.

Eating plants is also cheaper, especially if you can buy in bulk, spend some time reading recipes and learn to cook. Most plant foods, oats, beans, and such are fairly cheap, especially at today's huge markets. Your children will be healthy, and they will miss less school, so you will miss less work. You won't pay the social price of obesity. You will save your fellow citizens and the government a lot of money by staying healthy.

Beans are a great source of protein, 30%, and they have complex carbohydrates as well as vitamins, minerals and phytochemicals. You could cook them on Sunday night and feed the family with them for the next three days, saving you a lot of time and money. Beans are slowly digested and a friend to diabetics, since the insulin rises very slowly. We buy $1 trillion worth of food a year but we spend $2.7 trillion a year on sickness.

Plant proteins are much healthier than animal proteins because they don't carry the chemicals, pesticides, poisons and cancer factors of animal proteins. Besides, think of the cruelty to animals.

I recommend eating plants that are full of vitamins, minerals and phytochemicals, foods of color, no more than about 20% animal products, carefully chosen, low fat and high-protein. Avoid sugar, which is a toxin. Avoid the "Evil Twin" fructose.

The Story of Fat

FAT IS A TRIGLYCERIDE. THREE fatty acid molecules and one glycerol molecule

- Not all fat is bad; we need to eat some **essential fatty acids** every day because they are not made by our body. Most of us have heard the term Omega-3 and Omega-6 and these are the important essential fatty acids that we need. Omega-3 fatty acids, found in wild fish, are anti-inflammatory.
- Mono unsaturated fats include olive and canola oil
- Unsaturated fats such as vegetable oils are anti-inflammatory
- Saturated fatty acids-grass fed animal meat, milk and dairy products-cause atherosclerosis
- Medium chain triglycerides-palm oil, coconut oil-are a good energy source, with some suggestion of atherosclerosis
- Omega-6 fatty acids-farm raised animals and fish- can cause atherosclerosis, insulin resistance, immune dysfunction, are pro-inflammatory.

Before living things developed a circulatory system, single cell essential fatty acids jumped from cell to cell and those are the omega-3 and omega-6 fatty acids. They are anti-inflammatory, and they are the communicating systems between 70 trillion cells, so you can see how important they are. Without them we would not exist. The good eicosanoids prevent blood clots, cause vasodilatation, reduce pain, reduce cell division, enhance immunity and improve brain function.

The bad eicosanoids, the Omega sixes, promote blood clotting, cause vasoconstriction, promote pain, promote cell division, depress the immune system, cause inflammation and mental depression.

So Omega-3s are anti-inflammatory and sources are fish oil, flaxseed, nuts and vegetables.

The good Omega-3s include ALA, EPA and DHA. Omega-6s include LA, AAA, GLA and DGLA.

The four foods of the apocalypse are trans fats, alcohol, fructose and branch-chained amino acids.

TRANS FATTY ACIDS

They are transformed by adding one hydrogen atom into vegetable oils. They cannot be properly metabolized by the liver and are a great threat to your health. They increase your low density LDL, the one that digs into your lining of your blood vessels to cause atherosclerosis, heart disease and strokes. A doughnut, for example, may be 35 to 40% trans fatty acids, a killer. One-reason restaurants and markets like these products is that they don't rot.

Feedlot animal meat including beef, pork, lamb, chicken, turkey and fish (when raised on a farm) are a source of the Omega-6, AA, arachnodinic acids, versus ocean fish which is full of the anti-inflammatory Omega-3; organic-raised animal meats have more Omega-3.

Fat is metabolically very active and produces some nasty chemicals. Abdominal fat is more dangerous than fat on your hips, since abdominal fat is in your liver, pancreas and bowel and not just under your skin. It's very metabolically active. About 25% of the people in this nation have infiltration of the liver by fat. It causes scarring of the liver and interferes with its function. The latter results in insulin resistance, diabetes and more; most people do not know that they have a fatty liver, they may even be of normal weight.

The shape of the body and where the fat is located make a difference. If you are apple-shaped, you are more likely to have fatty liver disease. Non-alcoholic fatty liver disease will be the most common cause of liver transplants in the future and not cirrhosis from alcoholism.

How can you tell if you're overweight? This is important to know because 80% of the people who are overweight have metabolic syndrome and will develop significant chronic diseases like heart disease, vascular disease, strokes, cancer, autoimmune disease and dementia. So prevention is critical.

There are a number of ways to tell if you're overweight besides the visual estimate:

- Neck measurement: This is not well known but is the most accurate, check tables on the Internet.
- BMI-body mass index: Check tables and books and Internet
- Dexa scan
- MRI or ultrasound
- Pelvic-umbilicus ratio measurement

By age 2, we have 90% of our fat cells. How much we will weigh at birth is a lot of genetics and parents' habits. Then during intrauterine development, the weight of the child will be determined a great deal by the pre- and pregnancy habits of the mother. Is she smoking, is she taking drugs, what is she eating? My daughter had a baby recently and I reminded her to eat a lot of vegetables during her pregnancy. My two-year-old grandson looks just great.

Foods with a lot of trans fatty acids include biscuits, cookies, cream, crackers, donuts, fried foods, margarine and potato chips.

Obesity in our children is due in great part to the industrialization of food, fast food restaurants, plus ever-increasing combinations of fat, salt and sugar being served to us. The government is part of the conspiracy because they support the price of fat, salt and sugar to make food cheaper so we buy more of it. It's a combination of the industry and the government. Chicken McNuggets have 39 ingredients, many of fat, salt and sugar; McDonalds then adds a spray so that they taste like chicken.

We are born with a taste for salt, sweet, bitterness and sour. We have no fat taste buds. You have to teach your child to eat fat. We have receptors for sugar throughout our mouth, tongue, hard palate and all the way down the esophagus.

Is the U.S. Department of Agriculture interested in your health? If you visit the USDA in Washington D.C., you would find a huge department at the center of town. If you wanted to visit the nutrition office, the one that worries about your health, you would have to take a subway ride under the Potomac River, then take a bus ride, then walk one-third of a mile and take an elevator to the seventh floor in a building at the edge of Alexandria, Virginia. This small office supposedly helps to promote and protect your health. Who do you think has the upper hand here: the food companies or government officials? Or you, the public?

Let's not kid each other, we the people are irrelevant. It's the industry lobby with its money and the guys with their hand out who keep themselves in office to get the nice pensions and the best healthcare policies in the country. We the people pay the price with a shorter lifespan and many chronic illnesses. We need restrictions on the salt, fat and sugar content of food. The least we could do is tax the fat, salt and sugar and apply the money to health care.

We spend $1 trillion a year on food, and $2.7 trillion on health care, or let's call it "sick care".

Sugar is our methadone; it gets us on a high very quickly and makes us feel great. It affects the serotonin and dopamine circuitry in the brain. Fat is the opiate, a smooth operator whose affect is less obvious but no less powerful.

The molecules make us feel great like amphetamines, narcotics, sex, gambling, alcohol and cigarettes. The brain chemistry is exactly the same. A lot of people say food is more addictive than cocaine. This has been proven on functional MRI scanners. Ice cream lights up the scanner like an A-bomb.

The Cargill Corporation makes 17 sweeteners, 40 types of salt, and 21 oils and fats.

In 1999 about 10 CEOs of the largest food producers and manufacturers met at a hotel to discuss the increasing obesity problem. They fully agreed it was there, and a reporter dug out the information although this meeting was supposed to be completely secret. The industry decided to do nothing about it and said, in essence, "we don't give a damn. It's only profits that count."

Fat is energy dense and is 9 calories per gram, versus sugar and protein, which are 4 calories a gram.

Cheese is the largest source of saturated fat. Cheese is generally 50 to 80% fat, and we consume 33 pounds of cheese a year, plus 133 pounds of sugar year.

Whole milk is 3% fat, and one glass of whole milk has 225 calories, 7.5 g of saturated fat. No mammals drink the milk of another mammal except humans. Of course, mother's milk is a healthy thing and newborn children should drink it because of the good essential fatty acids. Our brain is 50% Omega-3.

The Kraft food company hired Paula Dean to sell a lot of high-fat sugary foods and help make the nation sick. In particular, she used their cheese in 5,000 recipes, helping the company make millions. Little consideration was given to the health of the public.

I accidentally walked into Paula Dean's restaurant in Savannah, Georgia. I had never heard of her and I didn't look at the sign on the restaurant. The first thing I passed was the fried food line and remember using the words "they should burn this place down" based just on what I was seeing inside the restaurant, many obese people and very nasty food. I did not know where I had been until I told some of the nurses at home this story and they said, "oh you must have been at Paula Deans'." Can you just imagine the number of people who became obese and unhealthy because of the food she was selling and advertising? Have you noticed she developed type 2 diabetes a few years ago but didn't tell anyone for years? Isn't it strange that people are not upset about this?

Nonalcoholic fatty liver disease, NAFLD, is a huge problem in this nation, and many people don't know they have it. Unfortunately, a significant number of people of normal weight have fat in their liver. Usually, though, their triglycerides or CRP would be abnormal to give you a hint. Therefore, you should get your biometrics checked even if you are looking good, feeling good and of normal weight.

In summary, to know the distribution of your fats is important no matter what you weigh. Fat, salt and sugar are what's killing us, with sugar the king of all. If you are going to eat some animal products, always know where they came from and eat as low fat as you can. Remember even beef that has all visible fat removed is still 20 to 40% fat, so don't fool yourself. A lot of people think chicken is a healthy food and they're just dead wrong; even without skin, chicken is 20 to 30% fat unless specially prepared.

Sugar

SUGAR IS OUR COCAINE. WE are hardwired for sweets by evolution. All our survival instincts like sex and eating are attached by chemistry to pleasure. Sugar makes us feel great and is addictive.

Our taste buds for sugar are located throughout the mouth, tongue, hard palate, and soft palate and down the esophagus to the stomach and even beyond to the pancreas and bowel. Sugar receptors have been found throughout this region. The receptors are not located just on the tip of the tongue, as some people might want to make you think. We have taste for salt, sugar, bitter and sour, and appreciate the softness and palatability of fat although no receptors have been found for fat. It is thought that there is a sense of taste for meat products called umani. We have thousands of taste bud receptors for sugar and they're hooked to the brain, the pleasure center.

As you know sugar is in a lot of our drinks, causing at least one half of the obesity epidemic, and is an ingredient in 80% of all 60,000-food products. Our sugar comes from three products: cane sugar, sugar beets and corn.

Christopher Columbus brought sugar to the New World and it was planted in Santo Domingo. People in France realized you could extract sugar from beets during wartime and now it's grown that way all over the world. Beets were the main source of sugar around 1970. Then the Japanese invented high fructose corn syrup, HFCS, which is much sweeter and cheaper and became very popular in the industry quickly. One of the reasons that it's cheaper is because the U.S. government supports the price of corn.

Unfortunately, corn syrup is high in fructose, which is not metabolized in the bloodstream but metabolized in the liver and made into low density LDL, the one that doesn't float and burrows its way into the blood vessels, neural cells and so on; it also has a lot to do with arthritis and hypertension.

In the 1960s it was proven in lab rats that sugar is addictive. Graduate student Anthony Scalafani studied the effectiveness of sugar and fat with functional MRI scans. The brain just lit up. He published a paper in 1976 with experimental proof of food craving as an addiction.

In Philadelphia there is a place called the Monell Chemical Senses Center, which is supported 50% by the government and 50% by the food industry. Guess who has a lot of influence there? They found and discovered a blood protein that is on the taste buds for sugar. That's how they were able to trace the tremendous distribution of sugar taste buds throughout the mouth, esophagus and gut.

They also determined that children and African-Americans were particularly keen on foods that are salty and sweet. The marketing people have taken full advantage of that. Hypertension is particularly high in the African-American population, so salt intake turns out to be something they really have to watch. When I worked in Washington D.C. as a resident in neurosurgery, I treated a lot of brain hemorrhages from hypertension in the black population. I saw blood pressures that were so high that I've never seen again, fortunately.

At the Monell Institute, they proved that children were actually becoming addicted to sugar because they were developing a tolerance for sugar. In other words you had to keep on increasing the amount, just like a narcotic addict, to get the same effect.

It's the taste, the flavor, the sensation and the psychological satisfaction that they are looking for.

Babies are born with taste buds for sugar and it's based on their biology, it's based on evolution and it's important for the survival.

A man named Moscowitz from White Plains, New York, whose company dealt with product development related to food substances and chemicals, did his best work with sugar. He used mathematical calculations to create the biggest crave. Moscowitz worked on "optimal sensory linking." Hunger was found to be a poor driver of cravings. Emotional needs are more important.

Taste, aroma, appearance and texture are very important.

The convenience of fast food restaurants brought the fat and sugar chemicals to the forefront of the etiology of obesity. The "cocaine effect" of sugar is its mother and father. The king is sugar because of fructose. Convenient, fast and addictive, salt and sugar drive the car. That process has been experimentally, chemically and mathematically proven. Look at the result: America the land of obesity.

It all started at the beginning of the last century. John Harvey Kellogg took over a health facility in Battle Creek, Michigan. The popular diagnosis at that time was neurasthenia and he ran a 400-bed hospital or institute. He came back from a trip to Colorado with an idea to create a breakfast cereal from corn. His brother Will, the accountant, managed to figure out how to make the cereal sweeter and the rest is history.

Fat-laden breakfast foods of the 1900s were then replaced by the sugar-laden cereals of the 20th century and we've all seen the result. Kellogg was home to 108 brands of cereal, and he then developed his own company doing the same thing. Kellogg composed of the top players for a long time.

The FDA was in bed with these companies and didn't consider sugar as being a threat to our health.

Dr. Jean Mayer, a Harvard professor, called obesity the disease of civilization. He discovered that the desire to eat was controlled by the hypothalamus in the brain.

Advertising to small children by food companies became rampant. They outlawed it in European countries. We restricted it only up to age 11 after a long fight, but companies simply increased advertisements to teenagers, and sales were not affected much.

Robert Woodruff, the CEO of Coke, had two brilliant but deadly innovations. In 1927 he introduced Coke with its sugary drinks to the rest of the world; in World War II any soldier anywhere in the world could get a Coke for five cents. I suspect he addicted the whole bunch. He figured out how to get into people's emotions with sugar.

A man named Jeffrey Dunn became head of the South American division of Coke; in 2001 he visited Brazil looking for new territory. He was looking at poor neighborhoods for the potential of sales. He woke up and said" I'm not going to do this." He decided the company went too far. Guess what? He no longer worked for Coke after that trip.

The Coke and Pepsi war has sugar as its king, with coffee not far behind.

In 1981 Coca Cola switched to fructose corn syrup because it was cheaper and sweeter; when they studied their customer base they didn't speak about loyal customers but called them heavy users, like you speak about a drug addict.

Eighty percent of world sugar is consumed by 20% of the people.

Nestlé, Kraft, Coke and Pepsi, all decreased the size of the drinks for a while so they could charge less and increase sales, especially in countries like Brazil. It's called the elasticity of demand. I see it demonstrated at my gym and it works. They have 9,000 members where I work out, $10 a month, I compliment them every day. A lot of people are getting in shape there. What they don't realize, though, is exercise is only about 25% of it.

I noticed in the news that Mexico may be passing a law putting a 10% tax on sugars and soda and 8% on fast food. Hallelujah to that.

In 1964, a man named John Yudkin published a book in Britain called "Pure, White and Deadly." He also published countless papers on the biochemistry of sucrose. Remember sucrose is 50% glucose, 50% fructose. Fructose gives the sweetness, is metabolized by the liver and converted to low-density cholesterol, small LDL fragments that penetrate the blood vessels and cause atherosclerosis and a number of other illnesses. It's clearly a toxin and is associated with vascular disease, heart disease, strokes, and other inflammatory illnesses.

Ancel Keyes, an epidemiologist from Minnesota, invented the K rations used during the Second World War. However, people started to note that high-fat dishes were leading to a high rate of vascular disease. This resulted in a battle between the fat and sugar camp as to the cause of disease.

In 1970, Michael Brown and Joseph Goldstein in Dallas discovered the HDL, LDL cholesterol and described the LDL receptor. This was a very important discovery. They correlated LDL-cholesterol with coronary heart disease.

Then we followed through with a national low-fat diet recommendation and forgot about the sugar.

Sen. George McGovern appointed a reporter named Nick Mottern with no scientific background to research and write a paper called the" dietary goals for the US." He gathered information from the work of Mark Hegsted at Harvard, a nutritionist. The latter thought that saturated fat was the cause of our health problems. The USDA, the American Heart Association and the Society of Clinical Nutritionists all endorsed the document.

The industry responded with low-fat, high-sugar products and you can see the result. A very obese nation became worse.

The mistake was in assuming that all LDL was bad; it turns out there are two types of LDL, A and B. As already mentioned, the large floats in the blood vessel represent 80% of it. Of the small LDL, 20% is produced in the liver by glucose and fructose, not fat.

A nurse's health study followed 50,000 nurses that were post-menopausal and fed them a 30% fat diet versus 40% fat and they found no difference in the incidence of vascular disease. I've heard others say that they didn't drop it low enough and that's a justifiable criticism. Dr. Joel Fuhrman said they should've dropped to 20% and the results would have been different.

The food industry took the fat out. The food tasted like cardboard and they solved that problem quickly by adding a lot of sugar. Sales went up tremendously and the industry was very happy and the country became sick. Our federal government supported the price of corn, wheat and rye. In the 1990s more low-fiber and high-sugar foods were produced. The obesity epidemic was born.

Seemingly logical, well-meaning people who don't understand the biochemistry of food have made a lot of people sick and continue to do so.

Our bodies have not adjusted to all of this sugar, especially fructose, and it's killing us; we consume 60 pounds of fructose a year, 33 pounds of high-fat cheese, 150lbs. of sugar. We are sugar and fat loaded; nobody and our bodies are revolting.

It's become a public health problem and the government needs to act.

The Real Enemy

THE REAL ENEMY IN TYPE 2 diabetes is insulin resistance. Our body requires energy-ATP-adenosine triphosphate. It's a gasoline to run the machinery of our body. Some cells, muscles and neurons require a lot more energy than others. Sugar provides energy that comes from food, usually carbohydrates.

Food starts breaking down with the chemicals and saliva in your mouth with its enzymes. Enzymes and acids break it down further in the stomach and intestines and eventually it ends up as sugar and enters the bloodstream. Now the pancreas gets to work and figures out the level of energy needed in the body and secretes insulin. It secretes insulin according to what the level of blood sugar is. Its job is to open the door of the cell to let in the sugar that can be converted with oxygen to the energy molecule ATP. It locks onto receptors on the surface of the cell, of which there are thousands on every cell, and sends a message to the inside of the cell to open the door to let the sugar in. A messenger from inside the cells says open the door to sugar.

Insulin is a chemical messenger. It signals proteins called Glut-4 transporters, which rise to the cell membrane, where they grab onto glucose and take it inside.

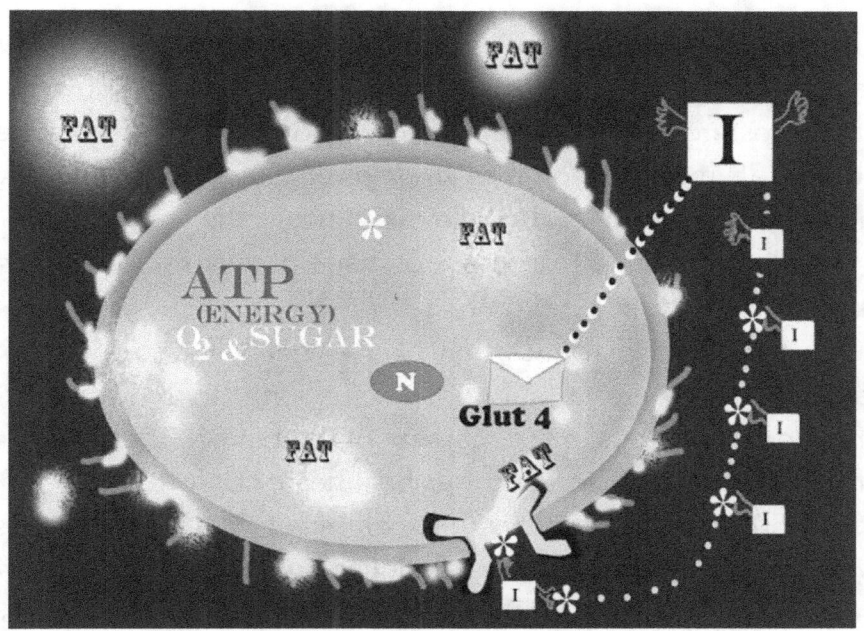

Insulin resistance occurs because fat makes your receptors sticky and insulin can't knock on the door of the cell.

The pancreas responds by sending out more insulin, more door knockers, sometimes to an excessive amount. Sugar eventually makes its way into the cell, but because the insulin level remains high in the blood, which is very damaging to the body, this can lead to inflammation, arteriosclerosis, and many other effects throughout the body. Insulin resistance is the first step in the development of type 2 diabetes. This explains why type 2 diabetics all have insulin resistance.

Over time, the pancreas wears out and the beta cells begin to die. Now we have type 1 diabetes also, which entails insulin shots. You don't make enough insulin now; you have to take it externally in addition to some oral medications.

Insulin resistance causes more trouble than diabetes, potentially leading to obesity, hypertension, high cholesterol, low-density cholesterol, strokes, heart attacks, and some forms of cancer. About 125 million people in the United States probably have metabolic syndrome and insulin resistance is the center of it.

Insulin resistance is in the crosshairs of syndrome X, a synonym for metabolic syndrome.

Over 90% of diabetics that I have met have no idea what causes it. Many are at fault in this situation: I think we medical providers need to take the majority of the blame. Then again all of us need to participate in our healthcare. Unfortunately, only about 50% of the diabetics are compliant with their provider. Who knows for sure where the fault lies but let's face it and try to fix it. Incidentally, I've written a book "Motivating to Wellness," which may help one make the necessary lifestyle changes.

About 75% of the people who have metabolic syndrome have no idea that they have it. Probably 25% have a fatty liver, a disease that is largely the cause of insulin resistance.

I generally make drawings for patients to teach them what insulin resistance is, see them back monthly if they wish, have them listen to CDs, have them watch DVDs that I've made and that seems to motivate them because they realize my heart is in it. Together, we all need to keep on trying.

One provider told me that the patients don't want to change. I think he's wrong and that and we just have to figure out what motivates each patient. Believe me, most people will eventually get the point and give it a shot. When you eat the right food, type 2 diabetes decreases or vanishes in about 60 days, 80 to 90% of the time. Dr. Franklin House wrote a book called "The 30 Day Miracle" and says he can do it in 30 days.

Dr. Raven from Stanford University has been the world leader in the study of insulin resistance. He discusses the relationship between insulin resistance, hypertension, obesity, high lipids, low-density LDL, metabolic syndrome, and insulin resistance syndrome, or syndrome X. About 50% of the people who have metabolic syndrome will develop type 2 diabetes. No one knows the exact percentage for sure.

When there is too much sugar circulating in the blood, it can clog up small blood vessels by several different methods. Sugar metabolism increases free radicals; sugar attaches to the proteins and can damage the blood vessels in the eyes, kidneys, brain and extremities, causing significant harm. When it comes to affecting the nerves, it can lead to diabetic neuropathy, a disease characterized by pain, numbness and weakness that can lead to loss of extremities including amputations. Symptoms will develop including burning, itching, numbness, pain and paralysis. The symptoms may be confused with spinal problems, ruptured disks and stenosis. The pain can be excruciating.

Much evidence indicates that there is a link between diabetes and hypertension and it is due to hyperinsulinemia. A state of cellular resistance to insulin action sets up the observed hyperinsulism. The reason for the association of insulin resistance and essential hypertension can be seen in at least four general types of mechanisms: sodium retention, sympathetic nervous system over-activity, disturbed membrane ion transport and perforation of vascular smooth muscle cells. Last, insulin, besides causing hypertension and obesity, is also known as atherogenic. It enhances cholesterol transport into arterial smooth muscle cells and increases endogenous lipid substances by the cells. Insulin stimulates production of various blood vessel growth factors.

Also, insulin resistance increases serum uric acid, which is a cause of hypertension.

In summary, insulin resistance appears to be a syndrome that is associated with the clustering of metabolic disorders, including non-insulin dependent diabetes, obesity, hypertension, cancer and atherosclerotic cardiovascular disease. These cytokines in abdominal and liver fat lead to insulin resistance. Probably 25% of Americans have non-alcoholic fatty liver disease and the majority of them don't know it.

About 20 to 30% of normal weight individuals have insulin resistance and metabolic syndrome. So if BMI is not the last word, CRP, liver function tests, MRI or ultrasound, homocysteine, lipid profile, especially low-density LDL, a two-hour glucose tolerance test which includes blood sugar are all important for diagnosis.

Millions of years ago living things, fish, amoeba, protozoa, microbes, communicated from cell to cell with eicosanoids, one-cell fatty acids. There was no blood system and we still have that communicating system in our body today.

When you get a paper cut, prostaglandins respond and cause redness and pain and the leukotrines command and produce the chemicals of inflammation. They direct your white cell army of Marines, and Navy.

Obesity is now considered an inflammatory disease because insulin resistance is an inflammatory process. It is caused by the fat, salt and sugar that we eat on a daily basis as well as smoking. At age 60, half of the people in the United States have at least one chronic disease: severe arthritis, heart disease, strokes, dementia, Parkinson's disease, and 100 million people with pre- and type 2 diabetes heading towards 150 million people.

The devil of the inflammatory story is AA, arachnid acid. It makes the prostaglandins and leukotrines.

It was discovered in the late 1800s that aspirin could block the inflammatory response by inhibiting that Cox one enzyme. It resulted in the Bayer aspirin, which helped a lot of people by stopping a lot of the inflammatory response in its tracks.

Can we stop inflammation before it starts? It turns out that aspirin stops the prostaglandin pathway but not the leukotriene pathway. It can help the problem but it can't cure it.

The problem is we get a great deal of AA in our Western diets. Farm-raised fish for example versus ocean fish. Dietary AA and heart disease, diabetes, cancer etc. have been connected in scientific studies.

Older people have increased levels of AA, which is part of the aging process; we are, indeed, rusting.

Some government supported super foods are actually making us sick! Let's look at salmon, for example. Great health food because of anti-inflammatories Omega 3s? Wrong. Ninety percent of our salmon today comes from a feedlot and not the ocean, fed by government supported fat and sugar.

Farm-fed salmon is full of AA, the pro-inflammatory chemical. Ocean fish live on algae, plants, sardines and not soybean products, carbon products, chicken litter as they have on aqua farms. Always ask your waiter where their fish came from, the ocean or feedlot. We can indeed change things if we do that enough.

Ocean salmon is full of EPA and DHA, the good eicosanoids. Remember these are the terms you want to remember for good supplements. A four-ounce farm-raised salmon can have up to 1,300 grams of AA. This has been scientifically studied. If you need scientific proof read the book called "Inflammation Nation" by Dr. Floyd H. Chilton, Ph.D.

Two fried eggs have 146 mg of AA and should be avoided. And just think of the cholesterol in the yolk. There are actually high levels of AA in lean turkey, and pork is even higher in AA.

So what is the anti-inflammatory diet?

Avoid animal meat, including farm-fed fish, and salt and sugar. Sugar is pro-inflammatory because it is a carbohydrate as well as a fat. The fructose in sugar is your real enemy because of its chemistry and metabolism. I recommend an 80% plant-based diet, with carefully selected lean meat. Get at least 30 minutes of exercise a day no matter what. You just have to commit to it until gets to be a habit. I also do some tai chi while I'm walking; it's automatic and also is now a habit. Exercise helps the metabolism, and greatly improves the chemistry of your body while reducing stress. Most of us use sugar as a narcotic to relieve the stress. I wouldn't overdo it in supplements but I generally recommend some vitamin D, Omega-3 and a multivitamin and that's about it. Don't overdo it in supplements because they also have side effects. You're much better off eating 100% whole grain, if not gluten sensitive, vegetables, foods with fiber, little animal products and some fruit. I also wrote "The Secret of the Non-diet" for further information.

Inflammation

OUR HEALTH IS BEING DESTROYED by the effects of out-of-control inflammation.

It's the toxic food we're eating and drinking.

The epidemic of inflammation is a bigger cause of disease then our genetic structure. The government is putting the majority of research money into gene research. But it's what we were eating and drinking that causes majority of our illnesses, yet we are devoting very few healthcare dollars to study that.

Being overweight, having metabolic syndrome and type 2 diabetes is the consequence of increasing insulin resistance in the blood. The cause of type 2 diabetes, which is all around us, are the evil twins" inflammation and insulin resistance.

Inflammation is the monkey on your back, and the mother and father of insulin resistance. If there were no inflammation, you wouldn't have insulin resistance, and the resultant diseases and illnesses brought on by that.

Dr. Mehmet Oz says," inflammation is the rusting of your arteries." Inflammation is a fire where you can't see the flames.

It remains hidden for many years until you run some tests, and then it might be too late.

The immune system involves your thymus, spleen, bone marrow, white blood cells —they are your Army, Navy, Air Force and Marines, which are supposed to win the war and bring you back to good health. This happens when you may have a local infection. But in your body it's an unending war, with your arteries and nerves involved with chronic infection because we continue to supply the body with toxic foods like salt and sugar. As Dr. Herbert Benson from Harvard would say, there is a doctor living within everyone's body, the immune system that knows how to repair things. We are attempting to repair the chronic inflammation but are causing a lot of damage in the process.

Your low density LDL infiltrates the interior walls of you arteries and capillaries; the inflammatory process with its macrophages jumps in to try to repair the problem and causes plaque formation instead. This causes arterial narrowing and can lead to trouble. The inflammatory process occurs throughout the body, and in the brain it can lead to dementia.

Eventually inflammation leads to vascular disease, strokes, heart attacks, glaucoma, arthritis, kidney disease, neuropathy etc., and it can inflame your 300,000 miles of capillary blood vessels.

The realization that the immune system plays a role in the onset of most major diseases has now been well proven. The immune system is a major killer stimulated by what we eat and what we do.

One million teenagers have metabolic syndrome based on inflammation. This speaks poorly of the future. Inflammation destroys the body by friendly fire. We are destroying our bodies by what we do or don't do. We're shooting ourselves in the head on a daily basis. Just look around you: Most people are totally unaware of what they are doing to themselves or they're just closing their eyes.

Our nation is dying from bad food. Oxidation is the process of aging. It's like trying new food with a decaying fruit like a banana. It makes your apple brown and its skin wrinkles. This is the aging process. Smoking is a cause of inflammation and we all know that smokers may look 20 years older than they really are.

Macrophages are powerful immune cells that are sent into the arterial walls and can cause thrombosis and in turn a heart attack.

Anything that causes inflammation will in turn cause insulin resistance, and anything that causes insulin resistance will cause inflammation. They are the evil twins.

We can easily identify inflammation from a sore throat, which is obvious, but the inflammation in our body can be hidden and turn into diseases and illnesses, resulting in chronic disease, disability and death.

The inflammation that drives obesity and chronic disease is invisible and doesn't hurt. It's a hidden smoldering fire created by **your immune system** that is trying to fight off bad food, sugar, fat and salt in processed food as well as smoking.

What triggers the inflammatory process?

Sugar is number one, refined carbohydrates, trans fats and too many Omega-6s from animal meets and plant oils. Also artificial sweeteners, high fructose corn syrup, food sensitivities, gut bacteria, genetic makeup, food additives and chemicals, meat produced by concentrated animal feeding organizations, fish grown in feedlots, as well as gluten.

Mounting evidence underscores the critical role that inflammation plays in the development of type 2 diabetes.

Dietary sugars and refined flours are the biggest triggers of inflammation. They cause insulin levels to spike and start a cascade of biochemical reactions that turn on our gene's chronic inflammation.

Lack of fiber, too many inflammatory Omega-6s and not enough Omega-3s, plus anti-inflammatory essential fats lead to the development of systemic inflammation throughout the body.

Food sensitivities and allergies also add to the problem. Many people have gluten sensitivity and not a true allergy but they get sick anyhow with many systemic type symptoms but it is not as deadly, unless they have celiac disease.

Many of the reactions and allergies are from a "leaky gut" created by proteins, byproducts of food digestion that leak through holes in the gut. This occurs much more commonly with the reaction to genetically modified new foods. They have no evolutionary history. Many foods have been genetically modified. Our bread is not what it used to be; it's more of a Franken food, a byproduct of industrial agriculture.

Early Diagnosis

THERE IS A LOT OF controversy here. Opinion frankly carries the day. Decades old double-blind studies of nutrition and eating habits are hard to find. Forty-four years of experience in the field should have some value.

Common sense is the king here.

The HRA, health risk assessment, should be number one. That should begin in childhood. Exactly what age? That would depend on family history or if the child has unusual early onset of obesity. If grandparents, siblings or mother or father have significant metabolic illnesses or death at a young age, then biometric, blood tests should be run as early as age 2. The rate of obesity is actually accelerating in the 2- to 6-year age range. The sooner you correct the problem, the easier it will be. Eating habits honestly become more difficult to correct the longer they have been there.

Blood work will be abnormal before obesity sets in, but not always. Children should have their weight and height checked at least once a year and more so with a strong family history. If both parents are overweight, then the child has a 70% chance of being overweight. If one parent has a weight problem, than it ought to run around 30 to 40%. Generally, many providers don't check the biometrics, the blood work of teenagers unless there is a strong family history of chronic disease. Personally, I think that is a mistake. Even if they have a normal BMI, teens should fill out a health risk assessment form and have their biometrics checked. After all we're looking to reduce the rate of this plague tremendously. In the long run it will save tremendous amount of illness and health care dollars.

You need to check the metabolism of the liver after a basic HRA assessment, including:

- NMR-lipid profile: It determines the particle size and number of LDL, HDL and triglycerides. Large amounts of small dense LDL is a sign of trouble. Even normal cholesterol won't tell the story. You need a low density LDL test. You should have fewer than 1,000 LDL particles and less than 500 small LDL particles.
- Liver enzyme test-AST, ALT, GGT-to assess fatty liver
- 2-hour glucose tolerance test
- Serum insulin and blood sugar (1-2 hours of fasting)
- Lipid profile
- Cholesterol-<150
- LDL-<70
- HDL-> 60-female
- HDL-> 50-male
- Triglycerides-<100
- Triglyceride/HDL ratio
- Total cholesterol/HDL ratio
- Hemoglobin A1c
- Gluten panel sensitivity test

An insulin response test is very important to catch early metabolic syndrome or type 2 diabetes,

This test measures your insulin and blood sugar at the same time. This will help providers catch the majority of metabolic diseases very early when it is much easier to correct them.

The test measures glucose and insulin levels after a 75 gram gross load. Your blood sugar can be normal but you insulin could be sky high. I saw this many times in my practice.

That is why diabesity, diabetes and obesity, is not diagnosed early in 90% of people who have it. You can see why this is so critical. Look at the tremendous amount of disease we misdiagnose.

If you have abnormal lab tests, they should be repeated at least every three months while you are taking corrective action. The provider should see you frequently, otherwise get a new provider or insist on more frequent tests.

To assess the severity of complications if you have abnormal metabolic test and it is clear you have a problem, then you need to get additional blood tests. If you would like to use the Internet, take advantage of Dr. Mark Hyman's excellent website. I also recommend his book "The Blood Sugar Solution." You can download it at www.bloodsugarsolution.drhyman.com.

If we are going to stop this epidemic, we need to start very early.

Not everyone would agree. If 20 to 40% of people with normal weight have abnormal biometric liver testing, then according to Dr. Mark Hyman, we need to do regular biometric testing. This is the future. It is a lot easier to take corrective action at a young age. If we miss disease for up to a decade, then that person is missing out on years of their life.

We spend $2.7 trillion on health care yearly; we could reduce this by $1 trillion if we take more early action. Right now we have "sick care."

Obese teenagers should be treated aggressively while we still have a chance at changing their habits.

Everyone should exercise at least 30 minutes per day.

Although we don't hear a lot of great things about the English health care system, they practice preventative healthcare big time. Almost all patients have their biometrics tested on a yearly basis because they have found it to be highly preventative. The doctor's offices are full of signs promoting wellness such as phone numbers to call for additional help. The family doctor gets paid more for keeping you well. You will notice when you travel in Europe that obesity is not much of a problem. When Europeans come here, they are shocked by the size of our population. We badly need to create a culture of wellness, and number one on that paradigm is that the patient must participate in his or her healthcare. In addition, providers need to participate by teaching every patient when the opportunity arises. For example, I have CDs, DVDs and TV shows and take the time to coach most patients in spite of a very busy schedule. I've been doing this for more than 30 years. I also write books and they're all on Amazon. The majorities are about wellness from every angle.

In summary I highly recommend really persistent, repeated health risk assessment and biometric testing as the best way to turn the United States healthcare crisis around

Prevention through Fitness

EXERCISE HAS BEEN PROVEN TO be a huge component of health since ancient times. Look at the Greek and Roman Coliseums. Athletes were worshiped.

We've been promoting it to the public for two centuries.

Hippocrates, a physician in the fourth century BC, placed a lot of emphasis on prevention of illness. He recognized that natural living was the road to good health and involved regular exercise.

It was called "hygiene," a Greek word for health, embracing all the activities relative to health over which a person has control.

So practicing good wellness habits is actually demonstrating your "hygiene" in Greek terms.

Hygiene has been narrowed to mean cleanliness, but for the most of our history it meant all the things you could do to insure vitality and health.

At the beginning of the Industrial Revolution, we became more sedentary and started doing less physical labor.

Time and time again, a poor city dweller was contrasted with a farmer. And the health statistics proved that. The stockbroker versus the farmer.

Health promoters since the 1800s recommended the system of exercise and diet.

In the 1830s a populist health reform movement was started by Sylvester Graham, a minister. It was called "Grahamism." He demonized alcohol and meat from animals. He is responsible for the Graham cracker and he also recommended a vegetarian diet.

Strenuous physical exercise was strongly recommended, running over walking.

Another movement in the later part of the 1800s was called" muscular Christianity."

It had a profound cultural impact, elevating building strength and endurance to an act of faith. It was considered a spiritual duty to stay healthy. By the end of the 1860s, he who neglected the body was considered to be committing a sin.

The German system of exercise called Turnin gymnastics was brought to the United States in the 1820s. This incorporated strength, bending and weightlifting including dumbbells, but was not popular.

Then the new gymnastics was brought forth called the Lewis system, a formal physical exercise promoted throughout the country. The Lewis system was rapidly adapted across the country in schools and colleges.

In the 1860s the country turned to the strength-building program of George Winship. After signing up for medical school at Harvard, he invented a system of weight machines and gave lectures all over the country focusing on strength and health; he started a weight lifting mania.

Dudley Allen Sgt. developed the Sgt. system of weight training, using full weight machines at Harvard. It was adapted by 250 colleges, 300 public school systems and 500 YMCAs. People got tired of machines and we started participating more in team sports. You can imagine, though, that left a lot of children behind and many are still left out today. Most of the country is watching things, sitting on a couch eating bad food and not participating.

In the 1900s we concentrated on infectious diseases because they caused most of our illnesses and deaths.

In World War I and in recent wars, about 50% of the recruits did not pass a physical. Actually about 75% of today's children are not physically fit.

As I sit here at Starbucks, a 250-300 pound gentleman is sitting across the table with a high calorie drink and eating sugary snacks. He had a big "C" on his shirt and I was tempted to ask what it stood for? Couch potato? This is not meant to be funny but unfortunately it's common around in my area; I would bet my tennis racket he has diabetes and his future is bleak.

In 1963 President John F. Kennedy took a step in the right direction by promoting the Council on Physical Fitness, which is still operating in most of the schools in the country.

Jack Lalane, "the Godfather of fitness," promoted physical fitness for more than 70 years. He died at age 96 having lived a full life without illness.

In addition to strength training, yoga, tai chi, Zumba dancing, walking, running and swimming are all great forms of exercise than can improve physical and mental fitness.

Planet Fitness where I work out daily should be congratulated. They dropped the price to $9.99 per month. So now almost anybody can afford to work out. Personally, I think this should be part of every insurance plan. The above facility where I work out has 9,000 members; I think 5 million in the country. It makes me smile every day.

Infectious diseases were the biggest cause of death in the 1800s and first half of the 1900s. But now we look at the complications of what we are eating, lack of exercise, stress and more; we have a 75% adult obesity rate, and a 30% children's obesity rate.

The majority of diseases such as type 2 diabetes, hypertension, half of the various types of cancer, autoimmune disease and stress can be avoided with proper eating, exercise, stress reduction and strength training. We could reduce all chronic diseases by 80% and probably save $1 trillion in healthcare costs. I spoke to a 4th year medical student yesterday and she said, "she had one hour of nutrition education in her four years of medical school. She'll be doctor and study pediatrics by July! How do you spell "pathetic", "sad"?

What do I recommend?

First I think you need a basic understanding of your risk factors from your healthcare provider.

Exercise should be done by children, causing it to become a habit. It can't just be e-mail, texting, TV and watching team sports. I'm now 77 years old and exercise 90 minutes every day, and I did so even as a child living in New York City in Central Park. I worked 44 years as a neurosurgeon day and night and still managed to find the time to exercise. Either get up early or go to bed late or figure something out that matches your situation, because it is critical to your health. Exercise improves your metabolism and helps you avoid those chronic diseases. Exercise will generally not cause that much weight loss, eating the right food is a better way to keep your weight under control. My father lived to be 89 years old, my mother 97; they did it with a fatty German deli diet but they worked hard and walked daily a lot and didn't smoke, and the food was organic.

Since ancient times, yoga, tai chi and chi gong have combined stretching, breathing techniques, meditation and visualization to promote good physical and mental health.

They guide individuals through a set of motions to improve strength, balance and self-confidence. Western countries usually include flexibility exercises as part of the strengthening and aerobic workout routines. I highly recommend that.

Flexibility is the extent to which certain tissues in the body can change safely and comfortably. Flexibility decreases with age.

Inactivity fosters "cross-links" or binding of the proteins that can close off muscles, tendons and ligaments. These cross-links are reversible.

A stretch of 15 seconds is adequate.

Following is a sample exercise routine:
- Five-minute warm-up
- Five minutes of stretching
- A few minutes of walking
- Five minutes of weightlifting
- 30 to 60 minutes of aerobic activity

Do this at least three times a week,

The health benefits of exercise for people at risk of developing or having diabetes include:
- Improves glycemic control
- Increases metabolism and promotes weight loss
- Reduces risk of metabolic syndrome
- Improves insulin sensitivity
- Improves blood pressure
- Inhibits diseases such as heart disease, strokes, cancer and autoimmune disease
- Reduces stress and depression
- Increases muscular strength and size
- Increase neuroplasticity (grow your brain)

Dr. Franklin House feels intermittent training is the key to increasing physical activity among sedentary Americans. It is non-continuous activity that incorporates active rest for a fraction of a minute of moderate activity. I do that all the time. Walk moderately fast followed by walking slow on the treadmill, for example, for at least five to 10 repetitions. This will improve your reserve of your heart. You make your body work a little, then you let it rest a little, then you make it work again and so on. You do this by exercising five heartbeats above your target heart rate and then five beats below your target heart rate. You don't stop the activity completely; you slow down enough to rest. For example, you jog, and then you walk. The added benefits of intermittent training include greater weight loss and body fat loss.

Energy for activity comes in two basic metabolic sources, oxygen metabolism and anaerobic muscle metabolism. Aerobic fitness is a large burst of energy in a short period of time; sprinting or heavy lifting would qualify. You may go into anaerobic metabolism within about three minutes of exercise. The intensity of the activity exceeds the ability of the heart and lungs to get oxygen to the muscles being worked. But what is the gold standard of health, fitness and well-being? It's your VO2 max that counts. Anaerobic activity uses glycogen, a form of sugar stored within muscle cells.

Find your target heart rate and use it to train. Subtract your age in years from 220, then take that number multiplied by .65 and that is your target heart rate. Your training zone will be five beats slower and five beats higher than your target heart rate.

Frankly, walking a mile a day five days a week, fast slow, fast slow, depending on ability, plus lifting reasonable weights for 10 to 15 minutes three times a week, preceded by five minutes of stretching is good enough for most people. If you are eating good food, you will live to be 100.

It's your HRA, health risk assessment, your biometrics, the blood tests, exercise history, and what type of food you eating that will determine your health most of the time. Certainly genes can play a role but generally they will not express themselves unless you have bad eating habits and challenge your evolutionary genetic history. Genes play at best a 10 to 15% role in overall health.

Remember your HRA and biometric tests and your exercise routine above all. Also, get that 2-hour glucose tolerance test and serum insulin and blood sugar at an early age and periodically repeat it. Good luck.

Teaching by Example

Kathleen Palyo DNP

"I CAN'T LOSE WEIGHT NO matter what I do." Day after day we hear our patients utter these words.

I used to be one of these people. Then I decided to change my life. I've lost 150 pounds and kept those pounds off for more than eight years.

I'm a nurse practitioner in an endocrinology practice in Fort Wayne, Indiana. I started gaining weight when I began commuting from Angola, Indiana, to the Medical College of Ohio to pursue a master's degree in Nursing. I was always eating on the road, and the stress of balancing school and family drove me to put on even more pounds. The turning point: In January 1998, I traveled to Bangkok, Thailand, to present nursing research at a conference. When I saw a picture of myself at the conference, I was shocked to see how much weight I had gained over the previous 10 years.

At that time, I weighed almost 300 pounds, yet I never really saw myself as overweight. I decided it was time to drop the excess pounds; first, to avoid type 2 Diabetes (my mother passed away in 2000 from complications from diabetes), which is prevalent in my family, and second, to serve as an example for my patients.

How many of my patients would take diet and exercise advice from an overweight nurse practitioner?

I began my weight loss journey by walking 30 minutes a day, three days a week. I had more energy, but little weight came off. Then I changed my eating habits. I didn't follow a particular diet; instead, I used my health knowledge to guide my food choices. I gave up the Pop Tarts and donuts for breakfast and started eating more protein at every meal, such as omelets with cheese for breakfast, salad with chicken or tuna for lunch, and fish and chicken with lots of vegetables for supper. I reduced, not eliminated, starchy carbohydrates such as bread, potatoes and pasta. I included dessert occasionally but in much smaller portions than before.

I lost 30 pounds in the first 18 months. Next, I bought a treadmill and free weights so I could work out at home in the winter months. I added Pilates, and then joined Curves. With every pound gone, I felt better, which motivated me to continue -- even after I lost 125 pounds. I worked out 30 to 45 minutes four or five days a week. Despite setbacks and plateaus, my weight and body size continued to drop, albeit slowly.

After about five years, I had lost 100 pounds, just in time to celebrate my 50th birthday! I added ballroom dancing classes (a birthday gift from my staff) for more variety, and I lost two pants sizes and an additional 25 pounds after just eight weeks of instruction. Next, I started running, even though I had never been a runner before or participated in any sports. Since then, I have completed the Disney World and the Pittsburgh Marathons (26.2 miles!), the Indianapolis Mini Marathon twice (13.1 miles), the Warbird 10K (6.2 miles) and the Harvest Stompede (7 miles) in Traverse City, Michigan. I dropped my membership at Curves because I started losing too much weight. Who thought I would ever say that?

I recently turned 59, and I am healthier and more active than ever. I dropped from a size 24 to a size 6 despite going through menopause, a time when hormone imbalances cause woman to struggle with their weight. So far I haven't developed insulin resistance, let alone diabetes. Both my significant other and I are very health conscious, we don't deny ourselves anything; but we cook with healthy ingredients and use portion control. Yes, it takes planning and discipline, but the health rewards are worth it.

There is no secret to losing weight. It requires eating less and moving more. However, you must believe that you can do it. I carry a photo of when I was overweight, which I show to my patients. I tell them that if they believe in themselves, they can do it, too. I try to instill in my patients the confidence they need to succeed by starting with small goals of five to 10 pounds at a time. Once they realize that they can lose the weight, they develop a more positive attitude and usually can reach that goal.

In order to lose weight, you must develop an eating style and activity program that fits your life. My patients vary in age from young married couples with children at home to older adults with fewer family responsibilities. I recommend starting with small changes in daily meal planning, such as substituting healthy ingredients in their favorite meals, and encourage eating at least every four to five hours. I suggest that my patients eat three small meals daily with a snack or two, all within their financial means. We work on breakfast first, and then continue with lunch and dinner suggestions.

The addition of physical activity must be individualized based on age, work and home schedules, physical abilities, finances and family responsibilities. Exercise can be used as time with family or as a chance to be alone and get away from daily stress.

My patients start to enjoy the extra energy they get from being more active, which in turn spurs further weight loss.

Many of my endocrinology patients struggle with weight gain, especially menopausal women. I use my positive experiences with weight loss to advise them, and they are usually successful in their efforts. When one of my patients reaches a 100-pound weight loss goal, I like to treat them to dinner in celebration of their success: They are now in my 100 Club! I hope my own experience will inspire others to develop their own weight loss plan so they will have personal success stories to share with others.

Summary

IN THIS BOOK I TRY to drive the point home that early, repeated HRA evaluation and biometric testing (blood testing) starting as an infant, continued through adolescents, at middle age and senior years can prevent, reverse and cure a lot of the diseases and illnesses we are facing today.

This needs to be followed with public education, and we need to have nurses, nurse practitioners and physicians who know how to motivate the public. It is generally known among the medical profession that 50% of people do not participate in their health-care. The new revolution in healthcare must include" I must participate in my healthcare" as its top goal. We must select providers for their ability to teach others and how caring they are. Just handing someone a prescription will not do it, we must know our patients, and we must love our patients. Education and a hug will go further than 90% of the prescriptions.

When we know that 90% of diseases have to do what we are eating and that 90% of type 2 diabetes could be prevented or reversed by proper nutrition, what are we waiting for? It's my personal opinion that we could probably save $1 trillion a year. We are the least healthy nation in the world because of what we eat. Our evolutionary bodies are not used to this assault of fat salt and sugar.

The medical schools need to put teaching at the top of their list. I have begged them to give lectures there on prevention on a regular basis, but it's not on the national board examinations so my phone remains silent!

I would even add a gluten panel to the biometric testing. The rate of celiac disease diagnosis is much higher in other countries like Australia and Italy. We could avoid a lot of diseases and save a lot of healthcare costs by doing that.

Providers need to be adequately paid for preventing diseases and paid less if they don't.

As a patient, you have to make demands to your provider. Be sure your child goes to a provider who does HRA evaluation and biometric testing regularly. My friend Dr. Verula puts each child in front of a large computer screen and shows them their body mass index and the views of biometric testing with them, If the child is overweight, a conversation is started on what to do about it. He discusses the social aspects of the problem to the child and finds he can motivate them that way. Then he pulls in the parents and this discussion starts over again. Then they set goals, and he sees them and follows up within a reasonable amount of time to see if action has been taken. Incidentally, the doctor and I give cooking classes to parents and children.

The schools and our local government must all get involved in creating a culture of wellness. That way we may end up with a healthier nation, avoiding a lot of illness and suffering and at the same time improving our economy.

Prevention is my game. --Dr. Rudy

MORE RESOURCES FROM RUDY KACHMANN M.D.

Books:

The Golden Opportunity
Narcotics: The Highway To Hell
Pain: We Need a New Definition
The Fraud of Chronic Pain
Healing Cancer with The Power Of Your Mind
Live to Be 100 with a Sound Mind and Body
The Call of Life
The Fraud of Alzheimer's Disease (also available on DVD)
Nocebo: Placebo's Evil Twin (also available on DVD and CD)
The Secret of the Non Diet for Adults (also available on DVD and CD)
The Secret of the Non Diet for Children (also available on DVD and CD)
Kid Scripts: Just What the Doctor Ordered
The Psychology of Eating (also available on DVD and CD)
Reversing Type 2 Diabetes in 60 Days (also available on DVD and CD)
Welcome to Your Mind Body (also available on DVD and CD)
Secrets of Motivating Yourself to Wellness (also available on DVD and CD)

For more titles, visit www.amazon.com.

DVDs:

The Mind and Stress (also available on CD)
Living Healthier and Longer (also available on CD)

Chinese Medicine (also available on CD)
Acute and Chronic Pain (also available on CD)
Smoking Cessation (also available on CD)
True Vitality (DVD only)
Secrets of the Mind and Cancer (DVD only)

For more titles, visit www.amazon.com.